Copyright © 2017 Kyle J. Benson

All rights reserved. No part of this publication may be reproduced or distributed in any form or by any means, or stored in a database or retrieval system, without the prior written permission of the author, except where permitted by law.

Legal & Disclaimer

The information contained in this book is not designed to replace or take the place of any form of medication or professional medical advice. The information in this book has been provided for educational and entertainment purposes only.

The information contained in this book has been compiled from sources deemed reliable, and it is accurate to the best of the Author's knowledge. However, the Author cannot guarantee its accuracy and validity so cannot be held liable for any errors or omissions. Changes are periodically made to this book. You must consult your doctor or get professional medical advice before using any of the suggested remedies, techniques, or information in this book.

Upon using the information contained in this book, you agree to hold harmless the Author from and against any damages, costs and expenses, including any legal fees, potentially resulting from the application of any of the information provided by this guide. This disclaimer applies to any damages or injury caused by the use and application, whether directly or indirectly, of any advice or information presented, whether for breach of contract, tort, negligence, personal injury, criminal intent, or under any other cause of action.

You agree to accept all the risks of using the information presented inside this book. You need to consult a professional medical practitioner in order to ensure you are both able & healthy enough to participate in this program.

Contents

Introduction

Perhaps like me, you've also been struggling to lose weight, despite your best efforts to do so. Like me, you might have dealt with the issues of being overweight.

We all know how it's quite a struggle. However, I have managed to get over the hurdles of losing weight by incorporating healthy lifestyle changes and sticking to a balanced weight loss regimen. This is all possible thanks to my knowledge regarding the secrets of weight loss.

I used to weigh over 250 pounds, but now I have managed to bring it down to around 150 pounds. The reason why I created this book is to share with you my insights regarding weight loss, how I have managed to lose a significant amount of weight and the secrets I've uncovered, while I was on my weight loss regimen.

So, whether you decide to get into better shape as part of your New Year's resolution, or simply because you want to fit into that swimming suit or trunk come summer, there's never a better time to start shedding those extra pounds than now.

In this book, we're going to unveil 5 amazing weight loss secrets, which you might have never known before. We're going to figure out why a lot of people fail whenever they try to shed those extra pounds despite their best efforts, along with the things that you should know before you start with your weight loss routine. Lastly, we're going to read a few success stories from people, about how they were able to pull off such a feat.

At the end of this book, I hope you can apply my insights in your lifestyle. Not only will they help you gain the body you've always dreamed of, but they'll also transform you into a more wholesome and healthier individual.

Chapter 1: Why Lose Weight?

Before I engaged in a weight loss program, I often found myself thinking, "Why do I need to lose weight?", "What are the benefits I can get from losing weight?" and "Is it even worth it?". Those were the questions that kept boggling my mind. However, everything became a lot clearer to me, the moment I started putting an end to my issues with obesity.

I think that this question is a no-brainer, but the most obvious reason why you should lose weight is because it offers massive benefits to your health. Of course, there are a few other benefits that you can gain from losing weight. That's exactly what we're going to discuss on the next page.

The Benefits Of Losing Weight

If I were to tell you that you're at risk of heart failure, would you still remain in your sedentary lifestyle? This might be no longer surprising, but a report from the American Heart Association confirmed that 1 out of 5 people, who are at risk of heart attacks aren't really worried about improving their health.

If you are that 1 individual out of 5, you need to change your lifestyle and kick-start the changes that you want to make with your body immediately. But before that, let us first talk about the benefits you can get from losing weight:

1. It significantly reduces your risk of heart diseases

High levels of cholesterol within your body will cause body fats to stick in your arteries, which in turn leads to a higher risk of heart attack. Fortunately, by investing time in losing weight, you can get yourself out of the danger zone. According to a 2013 study by the American Heart Association, women who were struggling with obesity were able to decrease their total cholesterol scores over the course of two years, by simply losing as little as 10 percent of their total body weight. Aside from that, they were also able to benefit from lower levels of LDL (low-density lipoprotein) cholesterol, insulin and triglycerides, which also contribute to heart disease.

2. It helps improve your mood

Based on a preliminary study conducted by the University of Pennsylvania, obese adults who lose at least five percent of their total body weight were able to benefit from improved sleep and better moods over the course of six months. The improvement in mood might not be directly related to weight loss itself, but rather because they were able to log in 21.6 minutes more of sleep every night compared to just 1.2 minutes within a specific control group. By getting enough sleep, irritability and frustration can be avoided. Also, it helps regulate your appetite, thereby helping you to lose more weight in the process. Regardless of how you look at it, it's definitely a win-win situation.

3. You'll develop an improved taste

It might sound ridiculous, but losing weight actually helps you improve your taste. To be honest, I wasn't a fan of vegetables back then. I'd prefer eating ice creams, burgers, hotdogs, junk food, almost anything unhealthy – that habit resulted in me being overweight during my earlier years. However, as I finally decided to lose weight, I found out that my taste has somewhat improved. I started eating healthier foods like vegetables, fruits, whole grains, etc.

According to scientists, the reason behind it is that excess weight will influence the hormone levels throughout our body. This, in turn, affects the way our taste receptors relay information to the brain. Basically, if you are overweight, your taste sensitivity becomes lesser as your taste buds become dull with overuse. To get them up and running again, you need to start losing weight.

Bonus Chapter

<u>Before you continue… Claim Your FREE Bonus!</u>

To thank you for purchasing my ***End of Obesity*** eBook, I've specially prepared the bonus "Making Money Online" eBook for you.

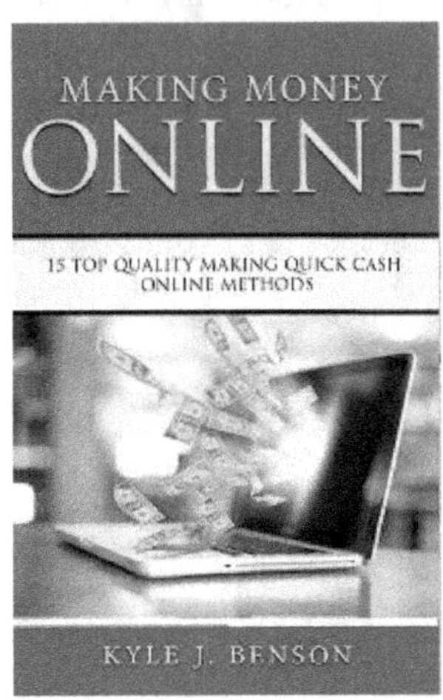

Inside, you will find:

- How To Make Extra Money As A Freelancer
- How To Make Extra Money With Your Design Skills
- How To Make Money From Online Advertising
- How To Sell Your Special Recipe Online Successfully
- How You Can Earn Money From Flipping Websites
- Discover The money Machine That is How-To Videos
- Make An Extra Buck Online By Just Doing Research
- 5 Websites Which Are Designed To Help You Earn Extra Income
- 4 Places Where You Can Sell Your Stuff Online and Make Money
- And Many More!

To download it, simply visit this URL: http://kylefreebook.gr8.com/ and put your email there, so I know which email address to send the eBook to.

Chapter 2: 5 Amazing Secrets About Weight Loss

Are you ready to uncover the secrets about weight loss? Before anything else, let me tell you this - these secrets that I'm about to tell you might not be as secret as they may seem. In fact, they are actually straightforward information. However, it is due to their straightforwardness that they are often overlooked and disregarded by most individuals, who are engaged in a weight loss regimen.

In spite of that, they hold a lot of power when it comes to losing weight. By learning about these secrets and incorporating them into your routine, you will be able to take the shortest route towards achieving the body that you've always dreamed of.

Also, along with each secret, we're going to discuss why most people have failed to follow through, along with a few success stories from individuals, who were able to gain successful results from each of these secrets.

At the end of each secret, you might be able to realize what you could have done wrong with your weight loss progress and figure out why yours has been awfully slow.

Now, let's start with the very first secret which is …

Secret #1: Fat Plays An Important Part In Weight Loss

Your diet may have prompted you to eat less and move more. After all, as long as we eat fewer calories and increase the duration of our exercise, we can lose weight successfully, right? Wrong.

For many years, even decades, we've been forced to believe that the best way we can control calories and lose weight is by cutting fat from our diet. However, it's actually the other way around. According to David Ludwig, a researcher focusing on obesity and nutrition at Harvard University, the time and energy, which we spend on rigorous exercises and strict diet regimens, might be better spent on paying attention to the foods we eat, instead of how much we eat.

We know that it might seem counterintuitive; however, the trick here lies in eating the right kind of food that contains the right kind of fat. I'm not talking about saturated fat, which is available in high amounts in processed meats and trans fat, which is mostly obtained from desserts. Rather, I'm talking about good fats in the form of monounsaturated fatty acids. Where can you obtain such fat?

Fortunately, monounsaturated fatty acids can be easily obtained from foods like nuts, avocados, and fatty fish such as salmon. These fats are capable of helping your body burn more calories, while keeping you fuller longer. A simple snack consisting of a handful of nuts, or perhaps peanut butter spread on whole wheat crackers, is more than enough to make for a healthy and terrific snack.

Why Most People Fail?

One of the main reasons why people fail in their weight loss attempt is because they try so hard not to include fat in their diet. They have no clue about the benefits fat can offer, when it comes to losing weight. This is due to the totally flawed low/no-fat principle that was widely embraced by the bodybuilding community back then. Bodybuilders might have been able to succeed with their diets, due to their extreme dedication to hitting the gym. However, most of those who have conformed to low-fat diets ended up getting fatter instead.

What To Know Before Losing Weight

A low-fat diet isn't effective in the sense that it doesn't make your body more efficient at fat-burning. Low-fat diets increase the enzymatic machinery in your body, which in turn causes it to become more efficient at burning carbohydrates instead.

Low-fat diets can also negatively impact the production of adipokines. In case you're wondering, adipokines are hormones that are produced from your fat cells. One particular hormone, adiponectin, is a fat-burning hormone, which enhances your body's metabolism and your body's fat-burning rate. By engaging in a low-fat diet, you're also lowering your levels of adiponectin.

The benefits of eating healthy fats are amazing, but one of the best benefits might be its satiating effect. Eating a low-fat diet will leave you hungry most of the time. It's the type of diet that prohibits you from eating foods with high-fat content such as cheese, nuts and fatty fish.

On the other hand, eating a diet that involves healthy fat will leave you feeling full. As your consumed fat reaches the small intestine, it will then trigger the release of hormones, which include CCK and PYY. These hormones play a major role in leaving you feeling satiated. Hence, by being more satiated, you'll less likely eat snacks in between meals.

However, while it's true that fat is good for you and can help you lose weight in the process, it's still not calorie-free. Instead, it's the exact opposite. In spite of this, a lot of individuals still add too much fat to their diets without any second thoughts. Although consuming more fat – roughly around 20 to 35 percent of your total calories – can benefit you, such calories often add up too quickly, hence you need to be careful.

How To Succeed Using This Secret

A particular story tells about the success of a woman named Candy Spiegel, who was able to lose 77 pounds during her first year of the plan. Her secret? She incorporated more healthy fats into her diet. Basically, she lost fats by simply eating more fats.

At 45 years of age, she was prediabetic and weighed a total of 298 pounds! It seemed as though all hope was lost, until she discovered a new diet book by Prevention titled "The Fat Cell Solution" by David Ludwig. In the book, he described how all those carbs and sugar that we consume can prompt our bodies to store fat. As such, insulin goes on a roller coaster ride, eventually causing us to suffer from constant hunger pangs and unexpected weight gain.

After reading the book, Spiegel immediately went on to undergo a weight loss program. Her new weight loss program involved eating twice as many fats as carbohydrates and avoiding foods like flour, sugar and pasta. Then, she went on shopping for healthy animal protein and fresh vegetables, and started cooking healthier meals.

Her first few months were definitely not easy, but the effort was all worth it. She ended up losing a surprising 2 to 3 pounds every single week. She continued with her program until a year has passed, and she was able to cut her weight down to 221 pounds!

So what does Spiegel's success story mean to you?

It's actually simple. By incorporating fats into your diet, you'll be able to lose weight faster than the usual weight loss routine. However, you have to make sure they're healthy fats that come from healthy sources such as avocados, salmon, mackerel, nuts, full-fat yogurt and cheese, to mention a few.

By pairing this with regular exercise and a balanced diet, it'll be definitely quicker and easier for you to shed those extra pounds.

Secret #2: Dairy Is Actually Your Friend

One popular weight loss myth that's been going around for ages is that dairy can only sabotage your entire weight loss efforts. However, you might be surprised to find out that dairy can actually help you lose weight! According to research, if you have calcium deficiency, you might end up losing appetite control, which in turn leads to binge eating and therefore incites unexpected weight gain.

Moreover, the research also figured out that consuming dairy from sources like yogurt, milk and nonfat cheese can actually help you accelerate your weight loss compared to other sources of calcium. A study conducted at the University of Tennessee discovered that eating at least 3 helpings of dairy per day can significantly reduce fats in overweight subjects. Furthermore, as they limited their calorie consumption a bit and continued giving the subjects the same servings, they were able to exhibit accelerated weight loss.

However, what actually happens if you stop including dairy in your daily diet?

If you want to cut dairy from your weight loss regimen, you might want to think twice about it. Even though dairy products can add major calories when consumed in excess, there have been several studies that prove dairy can help promote and maintain a healthy body weight.

However, this will still depend on what you replace the milk with, in your diet in the event you want to go dairy-free.

Why Most People Fail?

In a typical weight loss regimen, the goal is to achieve a significant loss of fat tissue. However, a significant amount of lean tissue is also lost during the process. Due to this, most people who undergo weight loss regimens weren't able to gain the outcome they desired. This could also be the reason why most weight reduction programs only led to weight regain, in spite of an improved dietary and workout behavior.

The reason is because lean tissue, likewise known as muscle mass, is metabolically active. It means that it will keep your engine at full throttle even though you are at rest. These past few years, various research and studies were conducted to uncover the role of dairy and calcium in weight loss and maintenance. Various findings were able to conclude that they actually contribute to weight loss and retention of lean tissue.

There have been several trials conducted in humans that verified the connection between consuming dairy products and accelerated weight loss, when paired with an energy-restricted program. One particular study has examined the effects of diets containing protein and calcium from dairy products to weight loss.

Findings supported the theory that eating foods rich in protein and low-fat dairy was effective at expediting weight loss and lean muscle mass retention.

What To Know Before Losing Weight

Dairy is a nutrient powerhouse, which is chock-full of calcium, vitamin D, protein, healthy fat, magnesium, and vitamins B6 and B12 – each of which is essential for weight loss. They help improve your energy levels, promote healthy metabolism and even kick your cravings. Moreover, since it takes longer for your body to digest dairy than carbs, and it also triggers the release of powerful satiety hormones within your guts, you will feel fuller after each meal with the help of protein and fat.

As you stay fuller longer, you will be able to skip that extra snack and even avoid overeating during your next meal. According to a study conducted by the British Journal of Nutrition, a high-protein cheese snack, which has moderate fat content will help you eat less during your next meal and throughout the rest of the day.

However, aside from keeping your cravings and preventing you from overeating, the protein you can get from dairy is also essential for building muscles and improving your metabolism. One study by the Journal of Obesity found out that individuals who consume dairy on a regular basis were able to gain 1.3 more pounds of lean muscle than those who skip on a dairy diet. If you skimp on dairy consumption, you'll end up missing a lot of essential protein from your diet. However, by adding even just a cup of cottage cheese, you can consume up to 50% of your recommended daily allowance of essential muscle-building protein.

That said, which dairy food should you eat to lose weight?

In order to expedite your weight loss progress with the help of dairy products, you have to go for low-fat dairy products like skimmed or semi-skimmed milk along with yogurts that are low in fat content. You should also make sure not to cut out cheese from your diet. In fact, you can now find low-fat hard cheese such as Cheddar available in the market nowadays. Other types of cheese such as Feta and Edam also make better choices than standard Cheddar, considering their slightly lower fat content.

How much should you consume?

The ideal daily consumption should be three servings of dairy food each day. It means drinking one glass of skimmed milk, one small piece of low-fat cheese, and one small pot of low-fat yogurt. However, a diet that consists of dairy is only recommended for those overweight individuals aged 18-50 years of age, who are on an energy-restricted diet and not lactose-intolerant.

How To Succeed Using This Secret

A lot of people avoid the consumption of dairy products when following a weight loss program. However, they didn't realize that this is actually counterproductive. You have to keep in mind that including dairy products in your diet will help you benefit from stronger bones and reduce the risks of cancer and blood pressure, apart from their known benefits to weight management.

But how exactly do you add dairy to your diet? Here are some simple, yet healthy ways to do so:

- Add cheese to your meals. Not only will it make your food taste good, it will also help you to benefit from its significant serving of protein. In fact, even just half a cup can provide you 12 grams of protein! However, you need to make sure to go for real cheese instead of anything that has a "processed cheese product" on its label.

- If you enjoy drinking coffee, it can help if you make it a latte. Or, you can also go for other milk-based varieties or simply add milk into the mix.

- Choose yogurt for dessert or snack. One 7-ounce of this creamy treat can provide you up to 18 grams of protein. Aside from that, it also contains live active cultures, which are basically probiotics, good bacteria which are widely known for their benefits to the immune system, digestive system and overall health.

- Drink a warm glass of milk before you go to sleep.

- If you don't like drinking milk, you can instead go for kefir. Kefir has approximately 15 to 20 times more probiotics than yogurt, and people who are lactose-intolerant can enjoy kefir due to its lower lactose content. Aside from that, it's even known to lower cholesterol and have anti-carcinogenic properties.

Keep in mind; however, that as you engage in a dairy-based diet, you need to follow a reduced-calorie diet, to achieve an effective weight loss.

Secret #3: Fidgeting Actually Does Wonders

I know that it sounds ridiculous. After all, who would believe that the simple act of squirming, tapping and performing little movements all throughout the day can actually help you lose weight?

Well, according to one study, fidgeting can help you burn 350 calories or even more in a day! Additionally, another research shows that people who are naturally lean find ways to shed those extra calories they consumed through fidgeting, even subconsciously.

But how is it even possible?

Even when you fidget, you're essentially moving your body. This action requires energy, and as such, it burns calories. But before anything else, you need to take note that even as we sleep; our body still continues to burn calories, although the rate is at its lowest. Therefore, fidgeting helps increase body movement, which would mean that more calories are burned.

People who usually fidget are ideally leaner compared to their more sluggish counterparts. In fact, several studies have shown that fidgeters can burn up to 2,000 calories more than those who don't, even when they live in the same daily environment. However, the majority of people who are classified as "fidgeters" aren't actually conscious of the extra movement they're doing. They just tend to do it naturally.

If you're not naturally fidgety, there are a few things you can do in order to consciously add more movement into your daily activities.

Why Most People Fail?

Most obese individuals tend to sit for prolonged periods, while healthy ones have trouble sitting still and often spend at least two hours a day on their feet, according to studies.

This difference alone equates to roughly 350 calories a day, which can be more than enough to produce a significant weight loss of 30 to 40 pounds in a year, even without heading to the gym. Basically, the reason why most people fail is because they don't act more restless like the thin ones.

The distinction might be due to biological factors and a result of the levels of genetically determined brain chemicals that influence a person's tendency to fidget. It is the tendency to remain inactive that causes obesity, not the other way around, according to researchers.

According to a study conducted at the Mayo Clinic, the activity levels were inborn and not the outcome of a person's weight because they didn't change when the subjects were subjected to weight gains and losses in various phases of the study. To ensure that they monitor the participant's eating habits; the researchers prepared all the meals for weeks at a time and have the subjects pledge not to cheat. Around 20,000 meals were prepared all throughout the study.

What To Know Before Losing Weight

Minute acts like shaking your foot, clicking the pen and tapping a finger might sound rather annoying. However, all those tiny acts of fidgeting can actually do good to your body. Apart from allowing you to burn extra calories over time, those little movements might even counteract the effects of sitting for longer periods of time, according to the study.

Whether it's in your workplace or while watching your favorite show, you'd probably spend hours upon hours every day sitting. These prolonged periods of sitting can have serious health consequences, and a study even reported that inactivity is one of the riskiest things to do right after smoking.

How many calories can you burn as you fidget?

The number of calories you can burn will depend on your intensity, the types of activities you perform, the duration of your movement, the size of the muscle groups that do the fidgeting, and individual bodily aspects like weight, fitness level and muscle mass. It's actually possible to burn up to 350 extra calories in just one day with fidgeting.

If you adopt the habit of fidgeting to lose weight, you can actually experience a significant difference compared to when you're not fidgeting. Theoretically, if you can burn up to 350 calories each day by fidgeting, it would mean burning up to 109,500 extra calories in one year! Assuming that you don't eat any extra calories, it would mean you'll lose a whopping 31.2 pounds!

The problem with using fidgeting as a way to lose weight is that people seem to do this by way of nature rather than nurture. It means that some of us are programmed to have a chemical makeup, which causes a person to become more inclined to perform spontaneous physical activities.

One final explanation is that fidgeting is a person's behavioral coping mechanism for stress. This particular theory about fidgeting focuses on behaviors such as biting the hair or skin, likewise known as displacement behaviors. However, such behaviors were not associated with anxiety in general – they just occur during really stressful moments. Surprisingly, this effect was shown to be more prominent in men, who displayed twice the amount of displacement behaviors as compared to women.

How To Succeed Using This Secret

Even if you're not fidgety, you can actually act like one. Here are some ways you can squeeze in a few extra activities in your daily routine. They're not as hard as you might think. They are the following:

- Get up from your seat every hour and walk around your workplace. You might also want to do some stretches. Even though you can't really become a genetic fidgeter, it is possible for you to consciously behave like one with enough effort.

- At the office, walk towards your co-workers, if you have something to say instead of communicating through the phone or messenger.

- Don't immediately sit at your desk right after lunch. You might want to go out for a quick stroll instead. If it's convenient, having your lunch outside of your office can also help.

- Learn to use the stairs instead of elevators and escalators. You might not know this, but you can actually burn up to one calorie for each step you take.

- Refrain from slouching in your chair. Instead, try to maintain a straight and erect sitting posture.

- Walk while you attend to a call on your phone. If you have a 10-minute phone conversation, it also means you have 10 minutes of walking!

- Stretch your body every now and then, even if you're at work or at home.

- Move as many parts of your body as possible. Wiggle your toes and ankles; twiddle your thumbs, and more. Try to let as many muscles as possible function, to maximize your weight loss.

- When shopping in the mall, walk around the entire mall first. Take time to enjoy the scenery, and then do your shopping afterwards.

The key takeaway here is that moving offers you a whole world of benefits than just sitting around. Various aspects of your body such as health, fitness and weight control can all benefit from fidgeting.

Secret #4: Eating Chocolates Is Actually Beneficial

It turns out that unsweetened cocoa, likewise known as dark chocolate, is actually beneficial for losing weight. However, the trick is to go for chocolates that are heavy on cocoa but light on sugar. The antioxidants you can find from dark chocolate will help boost the health of your arteries and prevent you from getting fat deposits. When consumed moderately, it can also help expedite your weight loss progress.

According to a 2010 study, consuming a small dose of dark chocolate can help reduce the risks of stroke and heart attack by up to 40 percent!

An ounce of dark chocolate containing 70% to 85% cacao is chock-full of nutrition. However, it can be counterproductive for individuals who have to limit their consumption of energy. With approximately 170 calories, dark chocolate is a sweet treat that should be consumed moderately especially due to its 12.09 grams fat content.

Dark chocolate contains 3 types of fats - good fat, monounsaturated fat (oleic acid), and saturated fats namely palmitic and steric acid. Fortunately, these fats can't have a negative impact on your cholesterol levels and are regarded as healthy fat, thereby making them essential to those, who want to lose weight quickly and effectively. Dark chocolate also has a number of essential minerals such as calcium, zinc, iron, copper, manganese, magnesium and potassium.

Why Most People Fail?

The problem with most people upon hearing the benefits of incorporating dark chocolate into their diet is that they tend to over consume. This is true especially for those who crave sweets that much. Eating just an ounce of dark chocolate thrice a week is more than enough to help you with your weight loss progress. However, eating too much can actually give you the opposite.

First of all, despite dark chocolate having high amounts of monounsaturated fat, it also contains some saturated fats. The content is even higher in brands with milk in them, so you might want to avoid dairy-free versions due to this.

Second, despite having higher cocoa content compared to milk and white chocolates, dark chocolate still has processed sugar. For example, a 72% cocoa bar has around 24 grams of sugar for every 100 grams of serving. This means that a hundred gram serving can provide an adult female's daily recommended sugar intake while two-thirds for an adult male. This only means that if you consume more than that, you can instead gain weight.

Hence, if you want to take advantage of dark chocolates to lose weight, you need to consume it in moderation. Consuming beyond your daily recommended intake can have negative impacts on your weight loss progress.

What To Know Before Losing Weight

Before you incorporate dark chocolate into your diet, you need to know how it can actually help you to lose weight. Here a few reasons that explain the benefits of dark chocolate in weight loss:

1. It controls your appetite

It might sound a little counterintuitive, but if you want to gain control over your appetite, you have to indulge in your cravings. Most weight loss programs will advise you to cut back on sweets and sugary foods; however, just a small dose of dark chocolate every day can help you control your appetite.

2. It boosts your metabolism

According to a study at Queen Margaret University, dark chocolate actually affects carbohydrate and fat metabolism, particularly when it comes to how our body synthesizes fats. This, in return, reduces the absorption of carbohydrates and fats. Therefore, if you eat dark chocolate, you can feel full. However, you need to choose the right type of chocolate, particularly dark chocolate containing 70% cacao or more.

3. It keeps stress at bay

You might not believe it, but eating dark chocolate can actually help you get rid of stress, according to a study in the Journal of Proteome Research. Since stress triggers the production of cortisol, you can experience unwanted weight gains due to an increase in appetite and stress eating. If you are able to manage your stress, you can also control what you eat. When you eat dark chocolate, you can increase the levels of endorphin and serotonin in your brain, thus allowing you to reduce stress levels and gain a major mood boost.

4. It reduces body fat

This is possible due to the presence of certain flavanols found in chocolate. These are plant-based nutrients, which are more prevalent in dark chocolate as compared to milk chocolate. However, too much can be counterproductive, hence you need to limit your consumption. It's advised to purchase individually-wrapped pieces and consume just one or two every single day.

5. It encourages intense workouts

Dark chocolate contains anti-inflammatory components, and if you combined them with its rich magnesium supply, you might end up feeling less pain. As such, you'll be more encouraged to perform exercises. Eating one ounce of dark chocolate with at least 70% cacao along with one glass of red wine during the night may offer you pain relief. Don't worry about not being able to sleep though: one ounce of dark chocolate has only 23 mgs of caffeine.

How To Succeed Using This Secret

You might have developed the notion that eating chocolate and losing weight just don't go hand in hand. However, as seemingly absurd as it may seem, it's actually possible to lose weight while enjoying your dose of chocolates – as mentioned earlier. Now, the problem is how are you going to incorporate chocolate consumption into your diet? How will you use this secret to your own advantage?

I've created steps you need to follow to succeed in your weight loss program. They are the following:

- Treat yourself to a moderate amount of chocolate every day and do your best to stick to it. Setting boundaries can help with your weight loss progress. Most of you might need to stick to a certain calorie balance in order to shed extra weight, so make sure that some of those calories are from chocolates.

- Make sure to consume dark chocolate instead of milk chocolate. Aside from having lower calorie content than milk chocolate, dark chocolate is also known to be more filling. As a result, you will feel full and satisfied quickly, while eating less. According to a study conducted at the University of Copenhagen, people who were offered dark chocolate ate 15% less of the pizza given to them afterwards. It is due to dark chocolate's appetite-suppressing properties that make it ideal to those, who want to lose weight.

- And if that doesn't sound appealing to you, dark chocolate is also found to be good for your cardiac health due to the flavanols found in cocoa! Talk about hitting two birds with one stone.

- Make sure you include healthy foods in your diet, so that you can allocate enough calories for a chocolate consumption. Make it a habit to eat fruits and vegetables, along with lean protein and whole grains.

- Instead of going for a morning coffee, why not switch to a cup of low-fat hot cocoa instead? It won't make you feel nervous like a coffee does, and you'll have your first intake of chocolate in the morning.

- Keep in mind that you need to limit your consumption of chocolate, if you're on your weight loss program. Make sure to enjoy in moderation and cut any source of extra calories. Otherwise, you'll go back to square one, and all your efforts might end up being wasted.

Just remember that chocolate is a treat, and just like any other treats and desserts, make sure you don't overindulge.

Secret #5: Exercise Alone Just Won't Cut It

If there's one thing a personal trainer will tell you about how to lose weight, it's definitely by exercising regularly. This might come as a shocker, but exercise alone is not enough (and might even be ineffective) for losing weight. As a matter of fact, exercise accounts for only 3 percent, or even less, of a decrease in your total body weight. The worse thing is that exercise alone as a means of losing weight will only induce more hunger, which in turn offsets any progress you've made.

Exercise is no doubt a vital component of weight loss. However, without proper nutrition, it will become quite ineffective. In order to shed those extra pounds and keep them off, you need to pair your exercise routine with a balanced diet.

I actually learned this the hard way a few years ago. For years, I believed that I can shove anything into my mouth just because I was actively participating in extensive workout sessions. However, the more I exercised, the hungrier I became. This caused me to eat more, thus allowing me to gain even more weight instead of losing. In fact, I noticed a steady increase in my body weight and gained a pound within a year!

Thinking that it's okay to eat just about anything you want simply because you exercise regularly is counterproductive. Of course, physical activity has a ton of health benefits to offer, but not if you don't keep your eating habits in check.

Why Most People Fail?

Contrary to popular belief, exercise alone won't help you to lose weight, according to research. While physical activity is essential for improving your overall health and fitness levels, there is very little evidence supporting that it alone can thwart obesity.

The reason why most people failed to lose weight by exercise alone is due to the fact that as you increase your physical activity, you suffer increased levels of hunger, hence increasing your appetite. As a result, you compensate for the increase in hunger by eating more food. Therefore, with or without increasing the intensity of your exercise, controlling calorie intake still remains the key to lose or maintain your weight.

While physical activity can provide you a slew of benefits, there has been evidence pointing out that an increase in exercise intensity is often offset by an increase in calorie consumption. Unless you pair it with a balanced diet, you're most definitely going nowhere.

What To Know Before Losing Weight

It's true that you need to exercise regularly, if you want to maintain your weight. According to a study by the National Weight Control Registry, people who were able to shed extra pounds, exercise regularly as a way to avoid gaining those pounds back.

At a physiological level, weight gain and weight loss are all about the right consumption and expenditure of calories. It is for this reason you need to understand the basics of calories. In other words, if you eat fewer calories than you expend, you can lose weight. Meanwhile, if you eat more calories than you expend, you gain weight. Hence, if you want to lose one pound of extra weight, you have to create a 3,500 calorie deficit. This is possible through exercise and diet.

As you exercise, you stimulate your appetite, causing you to eat more than you normally would without working out. Most of us assume that spending more energy will require a higher calorie intake, but we tend to overestimate most of the time. In fact, if you exercise just for the sake of burning calories, there's a very low return on investment. For example, eating just three cookies will require you to walk more than 45 minutes, just to burn off those 300 calories you consumed.

Aside from that, the idea that engaging in physical activity can boost our metabolism and cause our body to consume calories quickly is exaggerated. According to a study in 2012, a group of anthropologists studied the metabolic rates, physical activity, and energy expenditure of a hunting tribe in Tanzania and compared their findings to that of an average Westerner. They found out that even though the Tanzania hunters engaged in more intense physical activities on a daily basis, their metabolic rates weren't any different. To conclude, active lifestyles don't necessarily mean you're protected against obesity, if your diet includes an increase in caloric intake.

It's actually calorie consumption that fuels obesity. However, we're not just talking about the numbers – we're talking about the source. Sugar calories, for example, are particularly bad. Yet the public still continues to believe that they can maintain a healthy weight by counting calories and engaging in regular exercise. The food and beverage industry is the main culprit that spread the false belief that obesity is mainly due to lack of exercise.

How To Succeed Using This Secret

As mentioned earlier, if you want to succeed in your weight loss program with the help of regular physical activity, you need to pair it with a balanced diet. Due to the increased rates of obesity in the US, most people are eager to lose weight and improve their overall health. As such, hitting the gym and sticking to a healthy, balanced diet is essential. Here are a few steps to help you:

1. Determine the number of calories you expend every day. You can use various calculators on the Internet, such as ExRx's estimated calorie calculator.

2. Reduce your overall calorie consumption by up to 20% of your maintenance calories. Each time you decrease your consumption of calories, you need to simultaneously increase your protein intake, to keep you satiated. But how much protein should you eat while on a caloric deficit? According to nutritionist Alan Aragon, you need to figure out your target body weight, and then convert that number into grams. For example, if you weigh 250 pounds and want to go down to 150 pounds, you have to consume at least 150 g of protein every single day.

3. After you have become comfortable with calorie counting, it's time to switch to macronutrient counting instead. By focusing on macronutrients instead of calories, you can disrupt the fact that you and other people translate regular exercise and eating into a similar currency: calories.

As what you might have noticed, the steps I've mentioned above have no mention of exercise. Although you shouldn't factor exercise into your caloric consumption or expenditure, you should still incorporate it into your daily life. Sure, weight loss can be achieved in the kitchen, but overall health can be achieved in the gym.

Therefore, you shouldn't drop exercise as a part of your weight loss program. It's still beneficial nonetheless, but it shouldn't be your main focus when you want to shed all those extra pounds.

Conclusion

Now that we've reached the end of this book, it's about time to rethink your weight loss strategy. Perhaps one of the reasons why your weight loss progress is slow and somewhat ineffective is because you follow the usual routines recommended by so-called "weight loss gurus".

While they might show you effective and promising results, most of them might even offer you a weight loss program that will only take you longer to complete. Worse is, you might not even lose that much weight at the end of the program.

The weight loss secrets we've discussed in this book aren't based on personal assumptions alone. All of them are proven and tested by countless research and studies conducted by professionals. Basically, they were all backed by research. Of course, I shared parts of my personal experience by following the said secrets as well. And so far, the results were overwhelming. I think it's safe to assume that following and incorporating these secrets into my weight loss regimen hastened my weight loss progress, thereby allowing me to lose weight quicker and easier compared to previous programs I've tried before.

As you incorporate these secrets, I hope you can find your way towards an effective and fulfilling weight loss. Best of luck!

Again do remember to download your free special bonus eBook at http://kylefreebook.gr8.com/ and put your email there, so I know which email address to send the eBook to.

-- Kyle J. Benson

Check Out Other Books

Go here to check out other related books that might interest you:

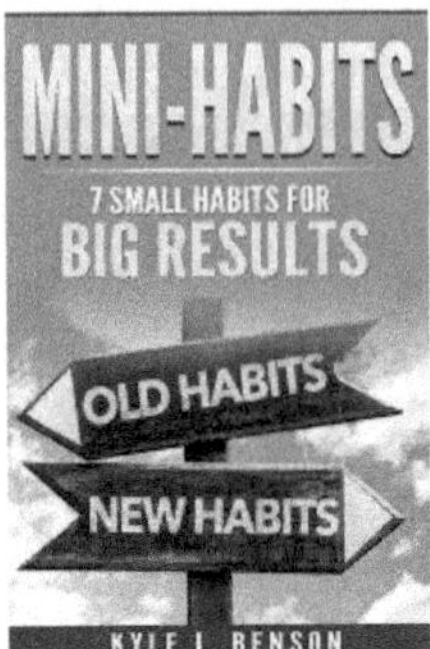

Mini-Habits: 7 Small Habits for Big Results
https://www.amazon.com/dp/B077FC1YGS

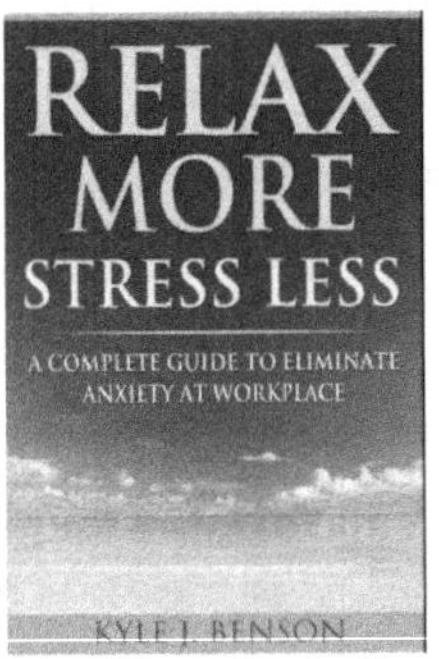

Relax More Stress Less
https://www.amazon.com/dp/B077M85X2S

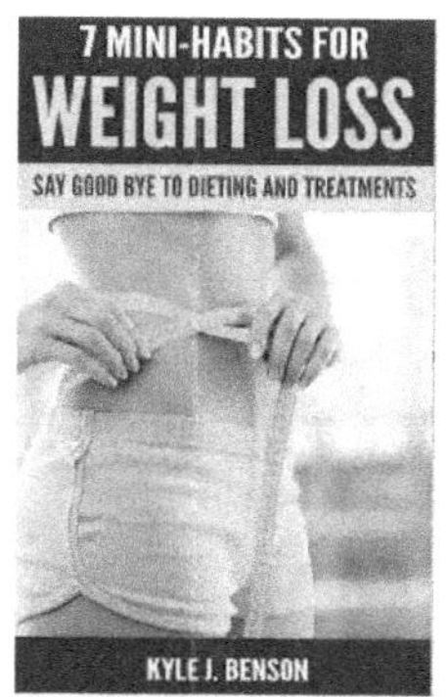

7 Mini-Habits for Weight Loss

https://www.amazon.com/dp/B077PN47M8

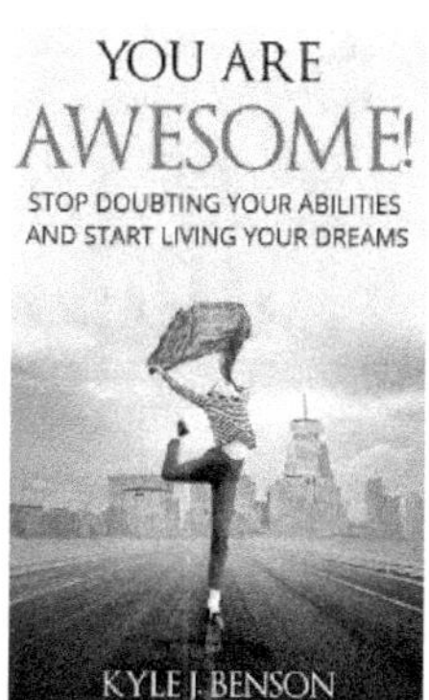

You Are Awesome!

https://www.amazon.com/dp/B077TGG7F7

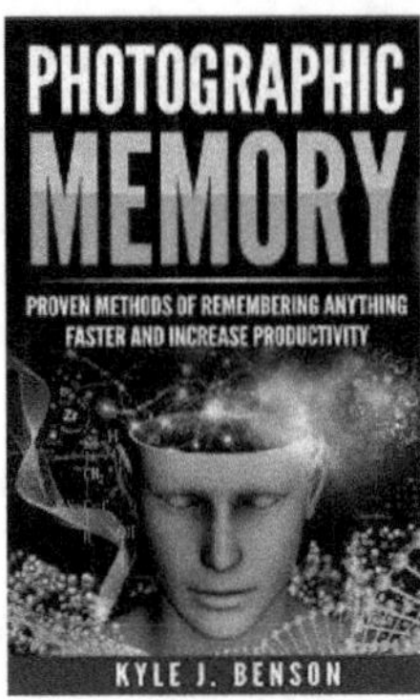

Photographic Memory

https://www.amazon.com/dp/B077VTXQ76

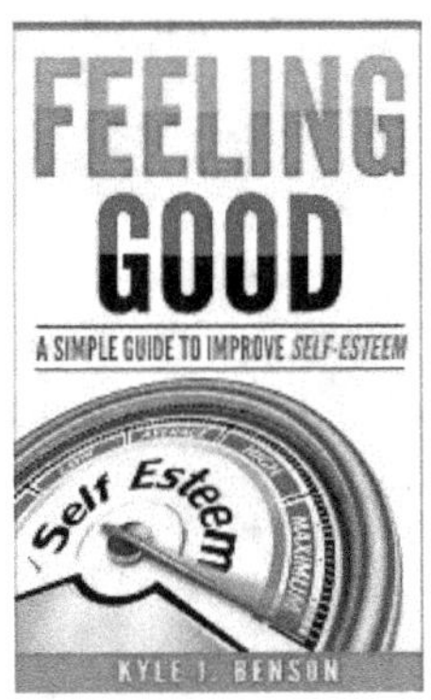

Feeling Good: A Simple Guide to Improve Self-Esteem

https://www.amazon.com/dp/B077P6CGZL